The PPE Handbook For Healthcare Facilities

Marjorie Quint-Bouzid

MPA, RN, NEA, BC

HCPro
a division of BLR

The PPE Handbook for Healthcare Facilities is published by HCPro, a division of BLR.

 5 4 3 2 1

Download the additional materials of this book at *www.hcpro.com/downloads/12520*

ISBN: 978-1-68308-097-8

HCPro provides information resources for the healthcare industry.

HCPro is not affiliated in any way with The Joint Commission, which owns the JCAHO and Joint Commission trademarks.

Marjorie Quint-Bouzid, MPA, RN, NEA, BC, Author
John Palmer, Editor
Erin Callahan, Vice President, Product Development & Content Strategy
Elizabeth Petersen, Executive Vice President, Healthcare
Matt Sharpe, Production Supervisor
Vincent Skyers, Design Services Director
Vicki McMahan, Sr. Graphic Designer
Sheryl Boutin, Layout/Graphic Design
Phillip Couch, Cover Designer

Advice given is general. Readers should consult professional counsel for specific legal, ethical, or clinical questions.

Arrangements can be made for quantity discounts. For more information, contact:

HCPro
100 Winners Circle, Suite 300
Brentwood, TN 37027
Telephone: 800-650-6787 or 781-639-1872
Fax: 800-785-9212
Email: *customerservice@hcpro.com*

Visit HCPro online at *www.hcpro.com* and *www.hcmarketplace.com*.

Contents

Acknowledgments

To the extent that this book is finally completed, I owe a debt of gratitude to the following persons for believing in me, encouraging me, and convincing me not to give up even after thinking about it many times. Having knowledge about a subject and the desire to impart that knowledge to colleagues and fellow healthcare workers does not easily translate to writing it in a coherent and readable manner. In my endeavor to complete this book, I learned this process is not as easy as one would think. Along the way it took many words of encouragement, many reminders to get moving, and many statements of "You can do this." This is why my sincerest gratitude for all the assistance I've had on the way and a heartfelt special thank you goes out to the following persons:

To Dell Harvell, RN extraordinaire, who helped to soothe my nerves when, at the ninth hour, I thought I could not pull this off. Not only did she speak positive affirmations, but she also helped me pull some key information together, which caused me to refocus. And that was just to complete an outline and Chapter 1. Thanks, Sis.

To Pamela Gailliard, RN, who, after listening to me share my desire to write a book about PPE as a way to share all the key lessons learned after rolling out a comprehensive PPE training program, conducting mock drills then having to re-educate, immediately responded "You can do it, no sweat." Thanks for believing in me and providing the encouragement in the early phases of this endeavor.

To Kevin Bussiere, RN, who served unofficially as a subject matter expert in matters pertaining to infection prevention and PPE dos and don'ts. I truly enjoyed our feedback sessions and your quick wit.

To my daughter Iman Bouzid, who incessantly reminded me that I could not give up, that I could complete this book, and that she believed in me. She continually reminded me to set aside time from my busy work schedule to continue with this project because she understood its importance. I find that impressive for a college student, as nagging and coaxing is supposed to be my job.

To my mother, Beverly Gordon, for her encouragement and never-failing optimism. She instilled a "can-do" attitude in me, which made it possible for me to press on when I did not feel like it.

To John Palmer, editor at HCPro, who took a chance on me and offered me the opportunity to author a training book. I sincerely thank you for the opportunity.

Marjorie Quint-Bouzid, MPA, RN, NEA, BC

Vice President Patient Care Services/Chief Nursing Officer

About the Author

Marjorie Quint-Bouzid, MPA, RN, NEA, BC, currently serves as vice president of nursing at Parkland Hospital and Health System in Dallas, Texas, and formerly served as the vice president of patient care services/chief nurse executive at Fort Washington Medical Center (FWMC).

Quint-Bouzid has over 30 years of experience as a registered nurse and more than 16 years of progressive experience in hospital administration. She has demonstrated experience in leading and managing successful teams. She has comprehensive knowledge of nursing issues, trends, healthcare regulations, and practice. She has advanced training in hospital emergency operations and has served as the hospital's emergency operations manager and as the incident commander during disaster situations. She frequently provides education and training on various safety topics such as safe environments, personal safety, and safety in the healthcare setting.

Quint-Bouzid holds a master's degree in public administration from Troy State University and a bachelor of science degree in nursing from D'Youville College. She has also attended the executive education program for nurse leaders from Wharton School of Business. She has been a sub-principal investigator on two research studies evaluating the effects of oxytocin on maternal fetal outcomes at birth and the effects of intentional caring behaviors on nurse retention. She lectures on topics related to patient and staff engagement and lateral violence in nursing.

Preface

After 30 years of a career in healthcare as a clinician and administrator, I wondered how to impart and share some of the things I've learned along the way. I'm at a juncture in my career at which I want to contribute to the greater body of knowledge.

Worker safety is of particular importance to me, as I strongly believe that the workforce must be healthy and protected from harm in order for the healthcare industry to thrive and fulfill its mission to society. For this reason, I find myself driven to assuming other duties as assigned at various levels of responsibility. I started out volunteering to be the unit-based safety coach, serving on a perinatal safety committee at several hospitals as a staff nurse. As a healthcare executive, I found myself leading several organizational safety councils, serving as the safety officer and the emergency preparedness manager. I was serving in this role when the Ebola crisis was in full swing. At the time, my organization had a relatively inexperienced occupational health nurse; similarly, so was the infection prevention practitioner. These would be the natural leaders of our Ebola response plan. Essentially, I looked at the current situation as a disaster and went into my emergency planner mode. The same principles of all-hazard preparedness for emergencies were applied to the situation: planning, mitigation, response, and recovery. All of my advanced training in emergency management for healthcare came to bear.

A multidisciplinary team of key stakeholders was quickly deployed, and within 10 hours the organization had its initial response plan. Of course, the devil is in the details, and the plan had to be tweaked and reworked almost every day for the following two weeks. Of course, I partnered with the state's Office of Preparedness and Response and local health departments to ensure we were using evidence-based practices and guidelines. During this time, I witnessed firsthand the sheer panic of healthcare workers when we discussed putting on and removing personal protective equipment (PPE). Reactions ranged from bravado, to tears, and to acceptance that this is an area of knowledge deficit. These reactions were demonstrated from every level of staff (nurses and doctors to environmental services workers). These are the personnel that we assumed were using these techniques on a daily basis when having to handle other more common forms of communicable diseases, such as H1N1, SARS, TB, and VRE. Conventional wisdom was that we would refresh the staff on which PPE to select and provide a brief update on the less frequently used PPE such as the respirators (N-95), and the training boxes would be checked off. In reality, we ended up having to conduct mass staff training on how to properly put on, take off, and dispose of PPE. Being on both sides, as the worker simply just trying to do my job and the manager wondering "why don't they just do their job correctly," I have a unique perspective on why healthcare worker safety and PPE remains a challenging topic.

I'm amazed how little intentional thought has been given to the topic of PPE by healthcare workers, given the nature of the work we do and the knowledge that in this line of work one could actually lose his or her life in the call of duty, at the very worst, or expose oneself or loved ones to contagious diseases. I have personally known several colleagues who have developed hepatitis C and tuberculosis disease due to workplace exposure. Each time I'm told someone I know has acquired an infectious disease, I momentarily become sad and question why as healthcare workers we are not more careful when it comes to taking seriously those things designed to keep us safer, such as proper hand hygiene practices and wearing appropriate protective equipment.

This idea came full circle for me during the 2014 Ebola virus disease (EVD) scare in the United States. Interestingly enough, when the news of the virus wreaking havoc in Africa started to come to our awareness in the United States, hospital administrators and practitioners intuitively knew they had to review their practices to protect their employees and other patients. However, many of my fellow administrators and staff voiced their belief that in our country we would better identify and contain the EVD because of our advanced knowledge of medicine and available resources. We listened to the news and felt sorry for those people over in Africa, but arguably we took no concerted steps to even bolster our healthcare workers' knowledge of and compliance with using PPE. I sat in meetings where comments were made to the effect that "after all, it must be the poor hand hygiene practice and lack of resources of those people" and so that was why the disease was spreading out of control. Others made comments such as "with our advanced knowledge of medicine in the U.S., we could keep the disease from spreading like it did in Africa."

Then it happened: We all saw the streaming images of men in moon suits transporting a person in an ambulance to a Dallas hospital in October 2014. Then we learned of the nurses and doctors stating they were not prepared for this kind of infectious pathogen in our healthcare system. We all know what happened shortly afterward. Panic and fear gripped the healthcare world, and then a calming realization that the whole notion of PPE and good safety practices will require more thorough and ongoing risk assessment, planning, preparation, and evaluation. The bottom line is that we are not as as prepared as we ought to be to handle even basic infection prevention. Approximately four years earlier than the Ebola crisis, the U.S. healthcare system thought it had bolstered up its knowledge and protocols around PPE when we experienced the H1N1, and then the severe acute respiratory syndrome (SARS) scare. How wrong we were.

The Purpose of This Book

This book is meant to serve as a quick guide for busy healthcare professionals when faced with the need to protect themselves from a potentially infectious organism in the throes of doing what they do best: caring for others.

While many resources are available from the Centers for Disease Control (CDC), Occupational Health and Safety Administration (OSHA), National Institute for Occupational Safety and Health (NIOSH), Institute of Medicine (IOM), Institute of Health Improvement (IHI), and many other state and local sources, they are lengthy, tend to be vague and open to interpretation, and are not consolidated under one umbrella.

There are more occasions than one would think where healthcare workers are not properly fitted for a lifesaving piece of equipment such as a respirator mask. This was painfully evident when a colleague of mine reported that during the Ebola scare her organization's protocol called for the physicians to wear a vented hood while the nurses were trained to wear an N-95 respirator mask. Neither of the groups underwent fit testing procedures. Furthermore, they were not monitored for compliance.

When I thought about putting together a pocket guide for the busy healthcare worker who wants to be compliant and do the right thing, I reached out to a longtime nursing instructor and asked her a simple question: "Why do healthcare workers struggle with complying with PPE?" She immediately responded that it's because the importance of PPE is usually not emphasized during a healthcare worker's training.

She went on to tell me that for the 11 years she's been a nursing instructor, she could not remember PPE selection and use as a topic on any course syllabus. It is not included in her orientation to new students.

This pocket guide is intended to bring all the pertinent information to the fingertips of the average healthcare worker in a clear and concise manner. It is meant to serve as a resource for clinical staff, administrators, healthcare educators, and practitioners. It is intended to not only discuss selection of PPE, but to also create a space for healthcare workers to review their beliefs and practices about PPE and address barriers to its effective use.

CHAPTER 1

Introduction: PPE for Healthcare Workers

The concept of personal protective equipment (PPE) for worker safety, like many other inventions, had its roots during wartime, then was applied to other hazardous civilian occupations such as firefighting, construction, and mining. The term often refers to protective clothing, helmets, goggles, and other garments that are worn to protect an individual from injuries.

One of the first large-scale and well-documented uses of PPE was respiratory protection against chemical warfare during World War I. The use of chemical gases shifted the dynamics of the war, and the use of respirators allowed troops to protect themselves from the toxic and harmful effects of the gas.

Leonardo da Vinci is credited not only with being a great painter, but also with inventing the first respirator during the 16th century. His idea was that soldiers could be protected from inhaling harmful dust and other toxic chemicals generated from weapons made of powder. With the advancement of technology and increasing demand, respirators became easier and less expensive to make. Over the years, they became less cumbersome, easier to wear and more durable, and thus more readily available for everyday workers. As with most safety advancements of our century, there were some regulatory pushes for worker safety that also aided in the proliferation of respirators and other PPE.

Federal agencies such as the Occupational Safety and Health Administration (OSHA) and the National Institute for Occupational Safety and Health (NIOSH) have developed standards that made respirators safer and more reliable and led to safety standardization and respirator fitting requirements.

As with respirators, other PPE initially developed to protect soldiers during combat evolved into what is now considered common practice for worker safety and protection. For instance, during the 4th century, the Japanese imagined the concept that metal plates strapped to the soldiers' and horses' torsos would prevent injuries during combat. With the industrial revolution, evolution of technology, and commercial development, the concept of protective armor is now manifested into disposable protective coveralls worn by healthcare workers to prevent contamination from chemical, biological, and physical hazards.

Another example of a type of PPE that evolved from combat use into an item of everyday personal protection is the helmet. Protecting the head is important because it contains the brain, which controls every aspect of our body and human functioning. The oldest known helmet was made out of leather or bronze and was used as far back as 900 B.C. In the early 1800s, shipbuilding workers would paint their hats in tar and cure them under the sun to solidify. When the hats hardened, they would be strong enough to protect people's heads from being struck by falling objects. Today, materials used in soldiers' helmets range from lightweight plastics to various types of synthetic fibers, once again demonstrating that technologic advancement and commercial research and development will continue to see protective equipment evolve.

Today in the United States, hard hats are mandatory when working on a construction site or in mining, and in any other workplace where strikes to the head from foreign objects, such as falling equipment, debris, and moving mechanical machinery are a hazard. In addition, secondary injuries such as slips, trips, and falls can also cause head injuries if the worker then strikes his or her head on an object. Despite its evolution in function, form, and availability, the main principles of PPE have not changed: to prevent hazards from entering or contacting workers' bodies, and to prevent hazardous materials attaching to workers' personal clothing from where it may subsequently enter their homes.

Evolution of PPE in Healthcare

Just like in other industries, modern PPE for healthcare workers evolved out of the need for occupational safety and health (protection of the worker) and as a means of infection prevention (protection of the patient). In short, PPE keeps both healthcare workers and patients safe from each other when exposures can be anticipated or expected.

Gloves for use in healthcare appeared in Germany around the 1760s when physicians used gloves made from sheep intestines for vaginal exams. In the 1840s, Charles Goodyear patented what he referred to as "vulcanized" rubber. This invention allowed development of gloves that were flexible enough to wear during surgery, and in the late 1890s, nurses at hospitals began wearing gloves on a routine basis when treating patients.

Surgical masks made from cotton gauze were originally worn by surgery staff in the early 1900s to prevent contamination of open surgical wounds. Around the same time, healthcare workers adopted the use of the same respirators used by soldiers to protect themselves from chemicals, firefighters to protect themselves from smoke, and miners to protect themselves from dust and gases. Historically, surgical masks were worn for airborne isolation precautions in hospitals when patients were known or suspected to be infected with pathogens spread by the airborne route of transmission.

Then, in 1990, new PPE guidelines for working with tuberculosis patients changed the game, when the CDC stated that surgical masks alone may not be effective in preventing the inhalation of droplet nuclei, and recommended the use of disposable particulate respirators. Later revisions of the guidelines based on further research led to NIOSH revising testing and certification requirements for all types of air-purifying respirators, as well as standards that require healthcare workers to wear respirators when working with patients with certain illnesses—and the training that employers are required to conduct.

Unlike the history of other forms of PPE, the use of goggles for eye protection is not clear. It's not a stretch to surmise that as blood sprays occurring during traumas and surgical procedures became a commonplace event, the need to protect the eyes from these body fluid sprays became important. It is thought that isolation gowns were likely born out of the common use of aprons and smocks in surgery and nursing—as a way to protect the wearer rather than the patient.

Why Is PPE Needed?

In the case of soldiers, they face extreme risks and hazards such as violent explosions, exposure to toxic chemicals, and biological hazards on a regular basis. To reduce the levels of danger, standard operating procedures or protocols are used in conjunction with protective equipment. Similarly, healthcare workers must follow safe work procedures, along with equipping themselves with the correct PPE. Although the equipment and procedures may not seem as extreme in comparison to combat protective equipment, the objective of occupational PPE and safe work procedures are the same: optimal safety when working in high-risk or hazardous conditions.

When used properly, PPE acts as a barrier between infectious materials such as viral and bacterial contaminants and your skin, mouth, nose, or eyes (mucous membranes). The barrier has the potential to block transmission of contaminants from blood, body fluids, or respiratory secretions.

Interestingly enough, the most important and least appropriately-used PPE is hand hygiene. We know human hands are one of the biggest culprits in transmitting pathogens to other parts of the body and to inanimate surfaces in the surrounding area and to other individuals. So it stands to reason that effective hand hygiene is the most basic of PPE. Hand hygiene and gloves are essential, both to protect the healthcare worker and to prevent the transmission to others.

Face cover, protective footwear, gowns or coveralls, and head cover are also considered essential to prevent transmission to healthcare workers. Not only is PPE effective in protecting the healthcare worker, but it also protects patients who are at high risk for contracting infections through a surgical procedure or patients who have compromised immune systems from being exposed to substances or potentially infectious material brought in by visitors and healthcare workers.

It is important to note that PPE alone will not fully protect you from acquiring an infection or transmitting an infection to another individual; however, we do know that when properly used with other infection control measures such as hand washing, use of alcohol-based hand sanitizers, and covering your cough and sneeze, these efforts dramatically reduce the spread of infection from one person to another.

CHAPTER 2

Types of PPE and Their Purpose

Worldwide, healthcare workers are aware that good, consistent practices of standard precautions save lives, yet studies continue to show marginal compliance with PPE usage. Personal protective equipment (PPE) for the healthcare worker is mainly geared toward providing protection from potential exposure to blood and body fluids to the skin and mucous membranes, as well as providing protection from contaminated air. In this chapter, you'll learn about some of the different types of PPE you will be exposed to in your career, and when they should be used.

Standard Precautions

For average healthcare workers, selection of PPE usually comes at a time when they are busy and just would like to know how to protect themselves. Remember, the foundation of all personal protection is that in uncertain situations where there is a risk of potential exposure, one should institute standard precautions (formerly known as universal precautions). In short, standard precautions cover the healthcare worker when there is a risk of the unknown.

The World Health Organization (WHO) defines "standard precautions" as measures taken to reduce the risk of transmission of bloodborne and other pathogens from both recognized and unrecognized sources. They are the basic level of infection control precautions that are to be used, as a minimum, in the care of all patients. It is widely known and accepted that the control of the spread of pathogens from the source is key to avoiding transmission. According to WHO, worldwide escalation of the use of standard precautions would reduce unnecessary risks associated with healthcare.

Basic protection

The Occupational Safety and Health Administration (OSHA) Bloodborne Pathogens standard (29 *CFR* 1910.130) mandates healthcare workers wear gloves in specific circumstances to reduce the risk of exposure to bloodborne pathogens.

Gloves are worn to provide a protective barrier and to prevent gross contamination of the hands when touching blood, body fluids, secretions, excretions, mucous membranes, and non-intact skin. Gloves are also worn to reduce the likelihood that microorganisms present on the hands of personnel will be transmitted to patients during invasive or other patient care procedures that involve touching a patient's mucous membranes and non-intact skin. Lastly, gloves are worn to reduce the likelihood that hands of personnel contaminated with microorganisms from a patient or an object such as a contaminated towel, clothing, or utensils will transmit these microorganisms to another patient.

Gloves help protect healthcare workers when they directly handle potentially infectious materials or when they believe they will come in contact with contaminated surfaces. Gloves can be made from vinyl, latex, or nitrile material. It should be noted that some healthcare workers are allergic to latex, and therefore, nitrile gloves should always be an option. As recent as May 2016, the FDA proposed a ban on powdered gloves, citing allergic reactions to the powder in some individuals.

It is important to remember that once contaminated, gloves can become a means of spreading infectious materials to healthcare workers, environmental surfaces, and others. Change gloves when heavily soiled, and never wash or reuse disposable gloves. Some basic tips to follow:

- ❑ *Work from clean to dirty.* Touch clean body sites or surfaces before you touch dirty or heavily contaminated areas.
- ❑ *Limit opportunities for touch contamination.* Avoid touching body parts, or adjusting glasses, rubbing your nose, touching your face, or any other actions that can cause you to unintentionally expose yourself to infectious agents that are on your gloved hands. In the same manner, touching environmental surfaces such as doorknobs, light switches, etc. unnecessarily can result in touch contamination.
- ❑ *Wash your hands after use.* Gloves do not replace the need for excellent hand washing or using an alcohol-based hand sanitizer.

Intermediate protection

Gowns are used in conjunction with standard precautions (gloves) to protect healthcare workers from the spread of infection or illness if they come in contact with potentially infectious liquid and solid material. Gowns may also be used to help prevent the wearer from contaminating vulnerable patients, such as those with weakened immune systems. Gowns are one part of an infection control strategy. The type of gown to be used should be based on the risk level below:

- ❑ **Level 1:** *Minimal risk*, to be used during basic care, standard isolation, cover gown for visitors, or in a standard medical unit
- ❑ **Level 2:** *Low risk*, to be used during blood draws, suturing, in the intensive care unit (ICU), or a pathology lab
- ❑ **Level 3:** *Moderate risk*, to be used during arterial blood draw, inserting an intravenous (IV) line, in the emergency room, or for trauma cases
- ❑ **Level 4:** *High risk*, to be used during long, fluid-intense procedures, surgery, or when pathogen resistance is needed or infectious diseases are suspected (non-airborne)

Advanced Protection: Full Barrier Protection

In the healthcare setting, certain diseases will require the caregiver to use full barrier protection. These diseases include but are not limited to severe acute respiratory syndrome (SARS), hemorrhagic diseases such as Ebola virus disease (EVD), and all known and suspected avian and pandemic influenza patients. Full barrier protection requires basic and intermediate protection, including:

- ❑ **Shoe covering.** Shoe covers provide a barrier against possible exposure to airborne organisms or contact with a contaminated environment.
- ❑ **Head covering.** Head covers protect the hair and scalp from possible contamination when sprays or airborne exposure is anticipated.

- **Eye and face protection.** Protecting the face requires use of a combination of protective interventions when contact with potentially infectious material is anticipated. The selection of facial PPE is determined by the isolation precautions required for the patient and/or the nature of the patient contact.
  - **Masks.** Surgical masks help to protect the nose and mouth from splattered body fluids (such as blood, respiratory secretions, vomit, feces, urine, amniotic fluid, etc.)
  - **Goggles.** Goggles protect the eyes, and thus should fit snugly over and around the eyes or personal prescription lenses. Eye protection must meet American National Standards Institute requirements (ANSI 287.1-1989). Goggles with anti-fog features will help maintain clarity of vision. Personal prescription lenses do not provide optimal eye protection and should not be used as a substitute for goggles.
  - **Face shields.** These protect the face, nose, mouth, and eyes, and are needed when the worker is irrigating a wound or suctioning copious secretions. A face shield can be used as a substitute to wearing a mask or goggles. The face shield should cover the forehead, extend below the chin, and wrap around the side of the face.

Respirators

Respirators filter the air before you inhale it to help protect you from microorganisms, including bacteria and many viruses. Respirators are approved by the CDC's National Institute for Occupational Safety and Health (NIOSH).

The types of respirators most commonly used in the healthcare setting are:

- ❑ **Surgical N-95 (N category at 95% efficiency).** This gives the protection of both a surgical or procedure mask, in addition to a filter that prevents the inhalation of small, infectious particles.
- ❑ **Powered air purifying respirator (PAPR).** This battery-operated respirator consists of a half- or full-face piece, breathing tube, blower, and particulate HEPA filter. These respirators also meet CDC guidelines for protection against tuberculosis (TB) exposure. They can be worn by persons whose facial hair or deformity would interfere with a mask-to-face seal.
- ❑ **Self-contained breathing apparatus respirator (SCBA).** These respirators, which include built-in oxygen sources, are not likely used by most healthcare workers, but are commonly used by emergency first responders in chemical, biological, radiological, and nuclear environments (CBRN).

References

For additional information on respirators, please see the following links:

www.cdc.gov/niosh/npptl/respirators/respsars.html

www.cdc.gov/niosh/99-143.html

www.cdc.gov/ni

CHAPTER 3

PPE Selection for Healthcare Workers

According to the CDC, standard precautions combine universal precautions and body-substance precautions for all patients regardless of diagnosis or possible infectious status. All contact with body fluids and secretions, except sweat, are to be avoided by healthcare workers. Also according to the CDC, transmission of infection within a hospital requires three elements: a source of infecting microorganisms, a susceptible host, and a means of transmission for the microorganism. So it stands to reason that protecting oneself from contact with the microorganism is the best possible defense in protecting the healthcare worker. A risk assessment is critical. Quick and simple risk assessments must be conducted by healthcare workers of all healthcare activities they will be participating in to determine the personal protection that is indicated.

Selecting Proper PPE

There are four major things you should bear in mind when selecting proper PPE:

- ❑ *Type of anticipated exposure*, such as splashes, sprays, or large volumes of blood or body fluids that might penetrate clothing.

- ❑ *Category of isolation precautions* a patient is on. See Chapter 2 for more about this.
- ❑ *Durability of the PPE for the task.* This will change depending on the task at hand. You'll need to decide, for example, whether a gown or apron you select needs to be fluid resistant, fluid-proof, or neither.
- ❑ *Fit.* We've all witnessed a colleague trying to work in gloves that are too large or a gown so big that it's falling off. If a piece of PPE doesn't fit you correctly, it won't protect you properly. It is the responsibility of the employer to demonstrate that the worker has been appropriately trained on how to put on gowns; likewise, it is the responsibility of the worker to follow instructions when wearing gowns.

Different Levels of PPE

In 1991, OSHA published the first Bloodborne Pathogens standard (29 *CFR* part 1910.1030), which required employers to set in place universal precautions and provide PPE to protect employees and patients. Several revisions have been made over the years, most notably the 2000 Needlestick Safety and Prevention Act, which added the requirement to help prevent injuries from unsafe sharps and disposal activities. As an employee, you should know the two tiers of precaution in hospitals or any other healthcare workplace.

Standard precautions

This is the basis of all infection control efforts in the healthcare setting. It always applies *regardless* of other precautions that are required. More recently, and as a result of the severe acute respiratory syndrome (SARS) epidemic, the concept of respiratory hygiene and cough etiquette has been added to standard precautions. SARS is caused by the coronavirus, the same virus that causes the common cold, and is spread through droplets in the air and close person-to-person contact. Healthcare workers must also consider that patients and family members with undiagnosed respiratory symptoms (runny nose, cough, congestion, productive secretions) could potentially be infectious.

Pro tip: Body fluids
Consider contact with all moist body substances, except for sweat, as potentially infectious.

Standard precautions consist of one or more of the following based on the risk of transmission and the risk of exposure. Also, see Chapter 2 for more information about standard precautions.

- ❑ Wash hands thoroughly before and after treating patients, and before entering or exiting any treatment room
- ❑ Wear gloves when touching blood, body fluids, secretions, excretions, and contaminated items
- ❑ Wear a face mask and eye protection (goggles, face shield) when there is anticipated contact with mucous membrane of the eyes, nose, and mouth during procedures likely to generate splashes or sprays of blood, body fluids, secretions, and excretions

- ❑ Gowns should be worn to protect clothing or exposed skin during procedures or patient care activities likely to generate splashes or sprays of blood, body fluid, secretions, and excretions

Pro tip: Gowns
DO NOT wear gowns for non-clinical reasons, such as warmth or aesthetics. Overuse of this PPE leads to normalization of deviance, as one is more likely to wear a gown inappropriately if it's not needed for protection from exposure.

Transmission-based precautions

Transmission-based precautions are for patients known or suspected to be infected by epidemiologically important pathogens spread by airborne or droplet transmission or by contact with dry skin or contaminated surfaces. Transmission-based precautions supplement standard precautions for an added level of protection when dealing with patients who have known or suspected colonization or infection of highly transmissible or epidemiologically important pathogens. These additional precautions are used when the route of transmission is not completely interrupted using standard precautions. In cases where the infection or disease can be transmitted via multiple routes, a combination of transmission-based precautions may be used. Whether used singly or in combination, they are always used in addition to standard precautions.

Why are transmission-based precautions used in hospitals? It's because agents and host factors are more difficult to control, and the interruption of the transfer of microorganisms is directed primarily at transmission.

Notes from the field

Having myself experienced being splashed with amniotic fluid in my eyes, I know the risk of not wearing proper PPE. During my orientation as a nurse, I was told to wear eye protection if I believed I would be splashed. Despite this, why would I believe I would ever be splashed after watching my peers (nurses and providers) forgo eye protection countless times during deliveries? After all, THEY never got splashed.

In actuality, what I saw was too many near-misses where nurses or providers jumped out of the way at the last minute, and then let out a sigh of relief that they did not get splashed in the face or the eyes. They apparently did not get the message, because during the very next delivery those same persons attended to, they did not think to use eye/face protection.

It's always been my intent to make the birth of a newborn look as normal as possible to parents and families, and walking in looking like I'm going into the room of an infectious patient doesn't sit well. I tend to use the least amount of PPE possible so as not to offend the family, but it wasn't until an incident where amniotic fluid flew across the room and landed in my right eye that I instantly knew I'd made an unsafe decision.

After my initial panic, I learned the patient was without any infectious pathogen. Most importantly, I learned another valuable lesson: Safety always comes first. You will do no good to your patients if you are not alive and well. As a hospital administrator, I tell each incoming new employee that they are to err on the side of safety always, and that means their safety, as well as that of their patients and colleagues.

There are basically three types of transmission-based precautions:

- ❑ Contact precautions (for diseases spread by direct or indirect contact)
- ❑ Droplet precautions (for diseases spread by large particles in the air)
- ❑ Airborne precautions (for diseases spread by small particles in the air)

Each type of precaution has some unique prevention steps that should be taken, but all have standard precautions as their foundation. We'll talk about each of them below.

Contact precautions

It is important to note that contact transmission is the most frequent mode of transmission of nosocomial or healthcare-acquired infections.

Contact precautions are used for patients that have an infection that can be spread by contact with the person's skin, mucous membranes, feces, vomit, urine, wound drainage, or other body fluids, or by contact with equipment or environmental surfaces that may be contaminated by the patient or by his/her secretions and excretions.

Examples of infections/conditions that are transmitted through direct or indirect contact include the following:

- ❑ Salmonella
- ❑ Scabies
- ❑ Shigella
- ❑ Pressure ulcers

In addition to standard precautions, adhere to the following PPE protocols:

- ❑ Wear a gown and gloves upon room entry of a patient on contact precautions. Use disposable single-use or patient-dedicated noncritical care equipment (such as blood pressure cuffs and stethoscopes).
- ❑ In addition to the measures above, perform hand hygiene using soap and water and consider use of a hypochlorite solution (e.g., bleach) for environmental cleaning.

Droplet precautions

Technically, droplet transmissions are a form of contact transmission. Droplet transmission is considered a separate route of transmission primarily because the mechanism of transfer of the pathogen to the host is different from either direct- or indirect-contact transmission.

The term “large particles” usually means particles measuring 5 micrometers (μm) or greater. Droplets are generated from the source person primarily during coughing, sneezing, and talking, and during the performance of certain procedures such as suctioning and bronchoscopy. Transmission occurs when droplets containing microorganisms generated from the infected person are propelled a short distance through the air and deposited on the host’s eyes, nasal tissues, or mouth. The general rule of thumb has been that droplets will travel about three feet from the source to the host. However, studies suggest that droplets from organisms such as smallpox and SARS can travel a distance of six feet or more from source to host. Therefore, the suggested distance of three feet is considered to be a recommendation rather than a mandate. As a result, distance should not be the only criteria used to decide whether or not the use of a mask is appropriate.

These precautions are used for patients that have an infection that can be spread through close respiratory or mucous membrane contact with respiratory secretions.

Examples of infections/conditions that require droplet precautions include the following:

- ❑ Influenza
- ❑ N. meningitidis (one of the causes of meningitis)
- ❑ Pertussis (also known as “whooping cough”)
- ❑ Rhinovirus (also known as the “common cold”)

In addition to standard precautions, observe the following PPE protocols:

- ❑ Wear a mask upon room entry of a patient on droplet precautions. A single patient room is preferred. If not available, spatial separation of more than 3 feet and drawing the curtain between beds is especially important.
- ❑ Patients on droplet precautions who must be transported outside of the room should wear a mask if tolerated and follow respiratory hygiene/cough etiquette.

Airborne precautions

Airborne transmission occurs by dissemination of either airborne droplet nuclei (small-particle residue of evaporated droplets containing microorganisms that remain suspended in the air for long periods of time) or dust particles containing the infectious agent. Microorganisms carried in this manner can be dispersed widely by air currents and may become inhaled by a susceptible host within the same room or over a longer distance from the source patient, depending on environmental factors; therefore, special air handling and ventilation such as an airborne infection isolation room are required to prevent airborne transmission. Examples of conditions or infections that require airborne precautions include the following:

- ❑ Measles
- ❑ Tuberculosis
- ❑ Varicella
- ❑ Rubella
- ❑ Mumps

In addition to standard precautions, observe the following PPE protocols:

- ❑ Place the patient immediately in an airborne infection isolation room.
- ❑ In addition to standard precautions, wear a NIOSH-certified fit-tested N-95 or higher level disposable respirator, if available, when caring for the patient; the respirator should be donned prior to room entry and removed after exiting the room.

- ❑ If substantial spraying of respiratory fluids is anticipated, gloves and gown as well as goggles or face shield should be worn. Instruct patient to wear a face mask when exiting the exam room, avoid coming into close contact with other patients, and practice respiratory hygiene and cough etiquette.

Pro tip: Risk assessment
Assess the risk of exposure to body substances or contaminated surfaces BEFORE any healthcare activity. *Make this a routine!*

CHAPTER 4

Proper PPE Procedures

This chapter will focus on providing you with the proper way of putting on, taking off, and disposing of personal protective equipment in order to minimize the risk of cross contamination of yourself, your colleagues, and other surfaces in the immediate patient care areas.

The proper selection of PPE is only the beginning of PPE compliance. One must put it on in the first place, but also in the proper sequence for maximum efficacy. The procedure to put on PPE is most commonly known as "donning;" likewise, the procedure of removal or taking off PPE is known as "doffing." For purposes of this training manual, the terms donning and doffing will be used. It is important to note that healthcare workers should only don or doff PPE for which they have had adequate training and are appropriately fitted for and medically cleared to use—as is the case when using respirators. Use of these pieces of equipment without prior training can compromise the safety and health of the worker, patients, and colleagues.

Please also see the end of this chapter for a handy CDC graphic you can use for your own reference.

Putting On (Donning) PPE

Considerations before donning any PPE

- ❑ Remove all jewelry, watches, and cell phones, and secure hair. Eyeglasses should be secured.
- ❑ Inspect all PPE before putting it on.
- ❑ Make sure you are well-hydrated, particularly if you are putting on extensive PPE, as is the case with planned or potential exposure to biological agents such as the Ebola virus.

Donning a gown

- ❑ Select the appropriate type and size—be sure it is an impervious disposable isolation gown. Although isolation gowns are generally the preferred PPE for most healthcare settings, aprons are occasionally used where limited contamination is anticipated. If contamination of the arms can be anticipated, you should select a gown. Gowns should fully cover the torso, fit comfortably over the body, and have long sleeves that fit snugly at the wrist. Clean gowns are generally used for isolation. Sterile gowns are only necessary for performing invasive procedures, such as inserting a central line.
- ❑ Unfold the gown and ensure the opening is in the back.
- ❑ Gowns should completely cover the torso from the neck to the knees, from the arms to the end of the wrists, and completely wrap around the back.

Pro tip: Fitting into your gown
When putting on a gown, first tie the straps in a bow, slip it over your head, then put arms through the gown. If the gown is too small to fully cover your torso, use two gowns. Put on the first gown with the opening in front and the second gown over the first with the opening in the back.

Donning a face mask

- ❑ Place over nose, mouth, and chin
- ❑ Fit flexible nose piece over nose bridge
- ❑ Secure on head with ties or elastic
- ❑ Adjust to fit

Putting on an N-95 respirator mask

- ❑ Select a fit-tested respirator. Most healthcare organizations use an N-95 mask. If your institution uses powered air purifying respirators (PAPR), then you must be properly fit-tested and trained in its use.
- ❑ Open the mask by separating the nose and chin piece.
- ❑ Once the mask is completely open, place it over chin. Stretch bands over back of head. Position bottom band behind the neck and below the ears, and the top band at or near the crown of the head.
- ❑ Press down on the mask around the nose piece and the contour of the face.

- ❑ Holding mask at the nosepiece, place one finger inside the mask on the malleable aluminum chin piece. Pull down gently so the mask is snug against the face.

Pro tip: Checking mask fit
To check fit, place both hands along edges of the mask and exhale. If air escapes around your nose, adjust the nosepiece. If air leaks at the mask edges, unfold or untwist the chin piece and repeat steps 4 and 5.

Donning a face shield/goggles

- ❑ Position the goggles over eyes and secure to the head using the headband or earpieces.
- ❑ Goggles should cover the eyes but not interfere with vision.
- ❑ Position face shield over face and secure with headband.
- ❑ Adjust to comfortable fit.

Donning gloves

- ❑ Select the correct type of gloves depending on the purpose of the use—and considering whether the person has allergies, as glove material can be vinyl, nitrile, or latex. They can be sterile or non-sterile. Determine if one or two pairs are needed.
- ❑ Select the glove size appropriate for comfort and dexterity.
- ❑ Be sure the cuffs of the gown are securely tucked under each glove, providing for a continuous barrier protection for your skin.

Pro tip: PPE order
Although it may be counterintuitive for the healthcare worker, gloves go on last when putting on PPE. Once gloves are on, limit opportunities for touch contamination (face, gown, mask, goggles, and other environmental surfaces in the patient's room). Change gloves if they become torn or heavily soiled, and never reuse disposable gloves.

Donning biological PPE

PPE used for biological agents is a bit more extensive, and is usually done with a partner, as in the "buddy system," to help avoid errors. Consider the following procedures:

- ❑ Put on boot covers first. If wearing coveralls, boot covers are worn under pant legs to prevent pooling of liquids between the coverall pant leg and upper band of boot cover. If you are wearing coveralls with integrated socks, you can omit this step.
- ❑ Apply surgical cap. (Be sure to cover ears for additional protection. Check with your facility for the head/neck cover product.)
- ❑ Apply surgical gown. (All ties should be properly secured with a simple bow.)
- ❑ Perform hand hygiene.
- ❑ Apply N-95 respirator.
- ❑ Seal mask to the face, ensuring straps are not crossed and are properly located at the crown of the head and base of the neck.
- ❑ Perform a fit check of the respirator, breathing deeply in and out, and feeling with your hands for any air leakage.

- ❑ Apply face shield. (It should fit over the surgical cap and N-95 straps. Ensure face shield and head cover overlap to protect the forehead.)
- ❑ Apply standard patient care gloves. Bring cuffs of gown over the glove cuff.
- ❑ Apply outer gloves (second pair) with extended cuffs. Make sure that the glove cuff covers the gown or coverall sleeve adequately to prevent exposure when providing patient care.
- ❑ To prevent the glove from rolling down, tape the glove to the gown sleeve, making sure to fold down a small edge of the end of the tape (for easier removal during doffing).
- ❑ Double-check by having your trained observer/buddy check the integrity of your PPE. After PPE is on, the healthcare worker should be able to fully extend arms, bend at the waist, and go through a range of motion adequate to comfortably perform patient care without becoming uncovered.

Pro tip: Taping PPE
During my Ebola PPE training, I witnessed many staff who stated they preferred to tape various PPE to prevent them from coming loose. Should you choose to do so, do not tape N-95 respirators to the hood of a protective coverall or other PPE, as this may interfere with proper fitting, thus rendering the respirator ineffective.

Taking Off (Doffing) PPE

Any time a healthcare worker believes or suspects contamination has occurred, or will occur, he or she should err on the side of safety and use extreme caution during the PPE removal process. It is very important to follow a specific sequence of steps to prevent accidentally transferring any contaminants from the PPE to yourself or to the environment. Safe and effective removal of PPE allows one to remove potentially infectious protective coverings without contaminating your clothing, skin, or mucous membranes. As with putting on PPE, the proper removal and disposal of contaminated PPE is essential. Removal can be challenging, but is essential in preventing inadvertent exposure to pathogens, which is why careful attention to the procedure is required.

Considerations before doffing any PPE

The following consideration must be given when removing PPE:

- ❑ Assume that any surface in the patient's room could be contaminated.
- ❑ It is considered best practice that all removal procedures be done with assistance, but particularly so when there is a risk of infection from biological agents.
- ❑ The face/eye protection, or respirator and inner gloves, are always the last items to be removed.
- ❑ All contaminated PPE must be isolated, contained, and disposed of in accordance with federal, state, and local regulations. Check your facility's policies and procedures.
- ❑ Anyone wearing prescription eyeglasses should make sure his or her glasses are not contaminated when he or she removes PPE.
- ❑ Ideally there should be a separate area for removal of PPE outside of the patient's room. If that is not possible, create a "hot zone" immediately outside of the patient's room. This

area is considered contaminated, and must be separate from the clean area used for putting on PPE.

Removal of PPE after potential or real exposure to biological agent (such as Ebola)

- ❑ All removal procedures must be under supervision by a trained observer/buddy.
- ❑ A trained observer/buddy should be available in the anteroom or immediately outside the patient's room just outside the established "hot zone" to supervise and assist, if needed, the PPE removal process.
- ❑ The observer should use a checklist to avoid forgetting any steps in the process; he or she should watch carefully for any breach in protocol.
- ❑ After removal of PPE, conduct another visual inspection of the PPE to observe for any tears, nicks, or visible contaminants. Disinfect any visible contamination with an approved disinfectant wipe. An EPA-registered disinfectant spray can be used on heavy contamination if permitted by your institution. Disinfect your outer gloves with an alcohol-based hand rub.

Taking off gloves

Remember the outside of your gloves are contaminated. If your hands become contaminated during the gown removal process, immediately perform hand hygiene by washing hands or using an alcohol-based hand sanitizer.

- ❑ Using a gloved hand (it is easier to begin by using your dominant hand), grasp the palm area of the other gloved hand (non-dominant hand) and peel off the first glove.
- ❑ Hold the removed glove in the gloved hand.
- ❑ Slide fingers of ungloved hand under remaining glove at wrist and peel off second glove over first glove.
- ❑ Discard the gloves in a waste container.

Taking off goggles or face shield

- ❑ Using ungloved hand, remove goggles or face shield by lifting head band or ear piece from the back of the head toward the front of the head.
- ❑ Discard in a waste container unless the goggles are reusable, then place in a designated container for cleaning.
- ❑ Follow your facility's cleaning procedure.

Taking off gowns

- ❑ Untie gown first at the neck then at the waist. Be careful not to touch the front of gown or sleeves when reaching for the ties.
- ❑ Hold the gown in between the center of the torso and pull gown away from body.
- ❑ Turn gown inside out and roll into a bundle, being careful to only touch the inside of the gown.
- ❑ Discard into a waste container.

Removal (doffing) of biological PPE

- ❑ If wearing an apron, break the strap behind your back, and then break the strap that secures the apron around your neck. Pull the apron away from your body, and then roll it inside-out. Discard the apron in the biohazardous waste container.
- ❑ Sit down on the chair designated as "dirty" to remove your boot covers. Grasp the heel of one cover and slowly pull it off your leg and foot. Avoid touching your scrubs and shoes. Dispose of the boot covering in the biohazardous waste container. Repeat with the other boot covering. Afterward, stand up, step away from the dirty chair, and disinfect your outer gloves.
- ❑ Remove the outer gloves by grasping the glove on one hand with the other hand. Grasping the exterior of the glove at the wrist, pull the glove off of your hand, with the contaminated exterior folded inside. Hold the removed glove in the double-gloved hand. Slide a single-gloved finger under the wristband of the remaining outer glove. Gently pull off the glove so that it is now inside-out, forming a bag for the other glove, and discard. Disinfect the inner pair of gloves.
- ❑ Remove the face shield. It is particularly important to avoid contamination of the eyes and mucous membranes when removing facial PPE. Tilt your head forward and lift the shield by the strap. Lift it above and away from your head without touching the shield itself, and discard it in the biohazardous waste container. Disinfect your gloves.

- ❑ Leaning forward, grasp the hood near the top and carefully pull it off and away from your head. Discard it in the biohazardous waste container, and disinfect your gloves.
- ❑ Remove your gown by first undoing the tie at the waist. The trained observer/buddy may assist you in undoing the tie at the neck and the back of the gown.
- ❑ Should your trained observer/buddy assist you in the removal of your equipment, he or she must disinfect his or her outer gloves with an alcohol-based hand rub immediately after contact with your PPE.
- ❑ Grasp the shoulder area and peel the gown away from your body, turning the gown inside-out and wrapping it into a bundle. Only the interior of the gown should remain visible. Discard the gown, and then disinfect your gloves.
- ❑ Remove the inner pair of gloves as described for the outer pair, taking precaution to avoid contaminating your bare hands. Use an alcohol-based hand rub for disinfection after taking off the gloves. Put on a new pair of gloves once your hands have dried.
- ❑ Remove the N-95 respirator. To minimize the possibility of contamination, avoid contact with the respirator itself, touching only the straps. Tilt your head forward, grab the strap that is around your neck, and lift it over your head, allowing it to hang freely. Then bring the top strap over your head and use it to remove the respirator from your face. Discard the respirator, then disinfect your gloves.

- ❑ Sit down on the designated clean chair and use disinfectant wipes to clean all external surfaces of your shoes. Disinfect your gloves.
- ❑ Remove the last set of gloves as described previously. Disinfect your hands with an alcohol-based hand rub.
- ❑ The trained observer should conduct a final inspection at this point to identify any contamination of your surgical scrubs. If there is contamination, an occupational safety and health coordinator should be informed immediately before you exit the PPE-removal area. The observer may now be contaminated and should always perform the same PPE-removal procedures as the healthcare worker before leaving the anteroom.

For more information, check out CDC guidelines at *www.cdc.gov/hai/pdfs/ppe/PPE-Sequence.pdf.*

Disposal of Used PPE

OSHA regulates disposal of infectious waste at the federal level and each individual state. While each individual state's laws closely match federal OSHA's laws, there are some states with more stringent requirements dictated by the particular state's environmental protection agency and department of health. Check with your facility's policies and procedures for the proper way to store and dispose of used PPE.

It remains the employer's responsibility to provide the appropriate disposal containers with appropriate labeling, and provide education and training to employees. In the same manner, employees have some responsibilities. OSHA 29 *CFR* 1910.1030(d)(3)

(viii) specifically states that it is the responsibility of the employee to dispose of protective clothing in an appropriately designated area or container for storage, washing, or decontamination. Infectious waste poses a significant risk for the transmission of infections, so it must be handled in a manner to mitigate risk of contamination to those handling the waste.

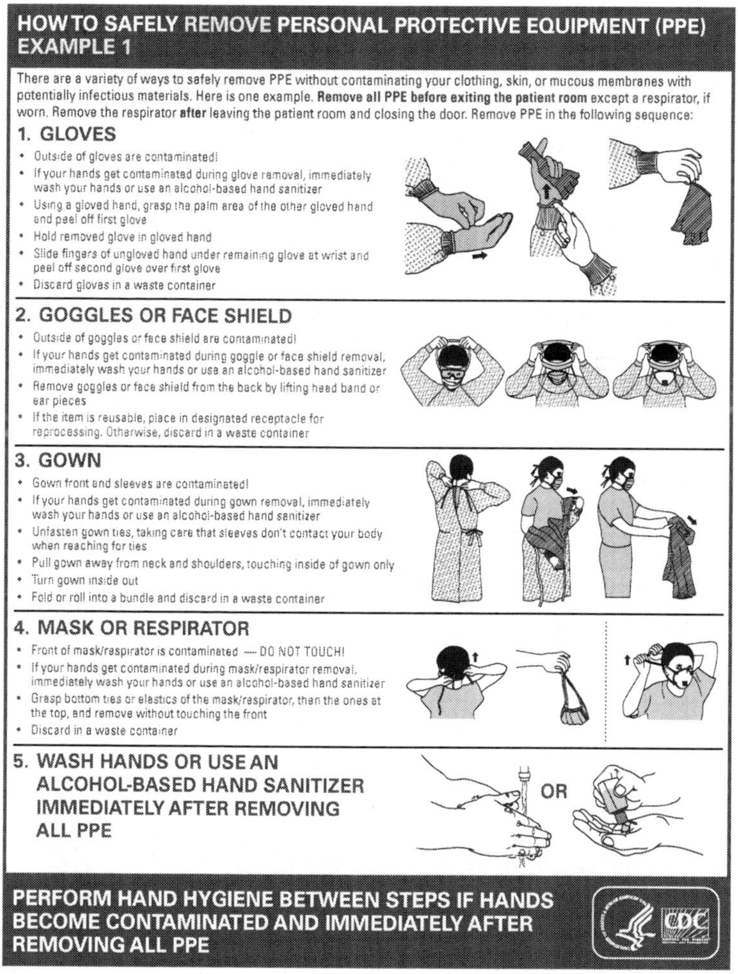

HOW TO SAFELY REMOVE PERSONAL PROTECTIVE EQUIPMENT (PPE) EXAMPLE 1

There are a variety of ways to safely remove PPE without contaminating your clothing, skin, or mucous membranes with potentially infectious materials. Here is one example. **Remove all PPE before exiting the patient room** except a respirator, if worn. Remove the respirator **after** leaving the patient room and closing the door. Remove PPE in the following sequence:

1. GLOVES

- Outside of gloves are contaminated!
- If your hands get contaminated during glove removal, immediately wash your hands or use an alcohol-based hand sanitizer
- Using a gloved hand, grasp the palm area of the other gloved hand and peel off first glove
- Hold removed glove in gloved hand
- Slide fingers of ungloved hand under remaining glove at wrist and peel off second glove over first glove
- Discard gloves in a waste container

2. GOGGLES OR FACE SHIELD

- Outside of goggles or face shield are contaminated!
- If your hands get contaminated during goggle or face shield removal, immediately wash your hands or use an alcohol-based hand sanitizer
- Remove goggles or face shield from the back by lifting head band or ear pieces
- If the item is reusable, place in designated receptacle for reprocessing. Otherwise, discard in a waste container

3. GOWN

- Gown front and sleeves are contaminated!
- If your hands get contaminated during gown removal, immediately wash your hands or use an alcohol-based hand sanitizer
- Unfasten gown ties, taking care that sleeves don't contact your body when reaching for ties
- Pull gown away from neck and shoulders, touching inside of gown only
- Turn gown inside out
- Fold or roll into a bundle and discard in a waste container

4. MASK OR RESPIRATOR

- Front of mask/respirator is contaminated — DO NOT TOUCH!
- If your hands get contaminated during mask/respirator removal, immediately wash your hands or use an alcohol-based hand sanitizer
- Grasp bottom ties or elastics of the mask/respirator, then the ones at the top, and remove without touching the front
- Discard in a waste container

5. WASH HANDS OR USE AN ALCOHOL-BASED HAND SANITIZER IMMEDIATELY AFTER REMOVING ALL PPE

OR

PERFORM HAND HYGIENE BETWEEN STEPS IF HANDS BECOME CONTAMINATED AND IMMEDIATELY AFTER REMOVING ALL PPE

CS250672-E

SEQUENCE FOR PUTTING ON PERSONAL PROTECTIVE EQUIPMENT (PPE)

The type of PPE used will vary based on the level of precautions required, such as standard and contact, droplet or airborne infection isolation precautions. The procedure for putting on and removing PPE should be tailored to the specific type of PPE.

1. GOWN

- Fully cover torso from neck to knees, arms to end of wrists, and wrap around the back
- Fasten in back of neck and waist

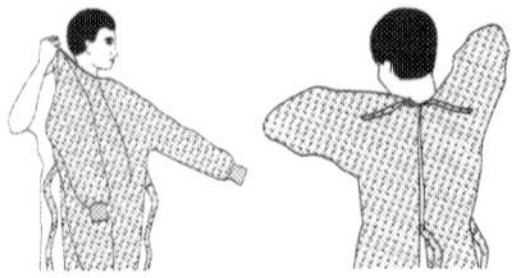

2. MASK OR RESPIRATOR

- Secure ties or elastic bands at middle of head and neck
- Fit flexible band to nose bridge
- Fit snug to face and below chin
- Fit-check respirator

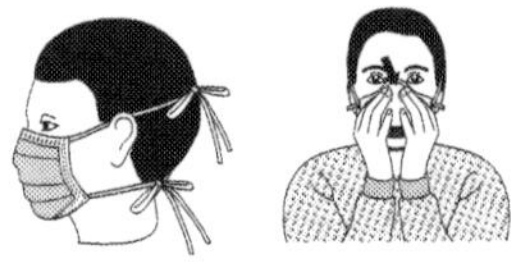

3. GOGGLES OR FACE SHIELD

- Place over face and eyes and adjust to fit

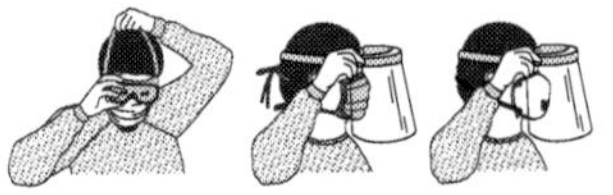

4. GLOVES

- Extend to cover wrist of isolation gown

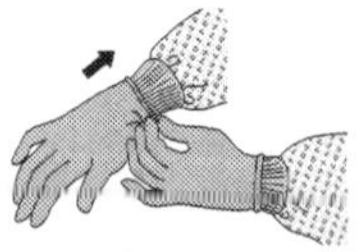

USE SAFE WORK PRACTICES TO PROTECT YOURSELF AND LIMIT THE SPREAD OF CONTAMINATION

- Keep hands away from face
- Limit surfaces touched
- Change gloves when torn or heavily contaminated
- Perform hand hygiene

CS250672-E

HOW TO SAFELY REMOVE PERSONAL PROTECTIVE EQUIPMENT (PPE) EXAMPLE 2

Here is another way to safely remove PPE without contaminating your clothing, skin, or mucous membranes with potentially infectious materials. **Remove all PPE before exiting the patient room** except a respirator, if worn. Remove the respirator **after** leaving the patient room and closing the door. Remove PPE in the following sequence:

1. GOWN AND GLOVES

- Gown front and sleeves and the outside of gloves are contaminated!
- If your hands get contaminated during gown or glove removal, immediately wash your hands or use an alcohol-based hand sanitizer
- Grasp the gown in the front and pull away from your body so that the ties break, touching outside of gown only with gloved hands
- While removing the gown, fold or roll the gown inside-out into a bundle
- As you are removing the gown, peel off your gloves at the same time, only touching the inside of the gloves and gown with your bare hands. Place the gown and gloves into a waste container

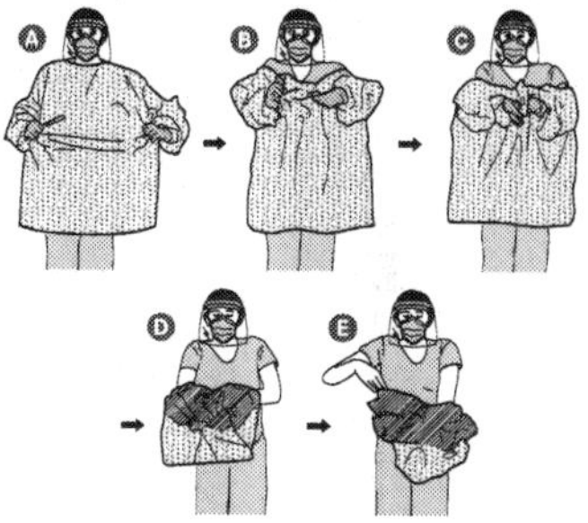

2. GOGGLES OR FACE SHIELD

- Outside of goggles or face shield are contaminated!
- If your hands get contaminated during goggle or face shield removal, immediately wash your hands or use an alcohol-based hand sanitizer
- Remove goggles or face shield from the back by lifting head band and without touching the front of the goggles or face shield
- If the item is reusable, place in designated receptacle for reprocessing. Otherwise, discard in a waste container

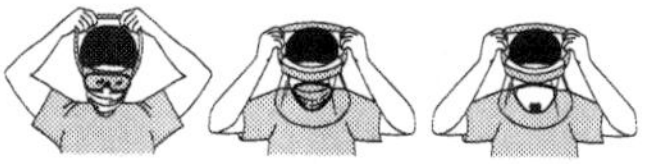

3. MASK OR RESPIRATOR

- Front of mask/respirator is contaminated — DO NOT TOUCH!
- If your hands get contaminated during mask/respirator removal, immediately wash your hands or use an alcohol-based hand sanitizer
- Grasp bottom ties or elastics of the mask/respirator, then the ones at the top, and remove without touching the front
- Discard in a waste container

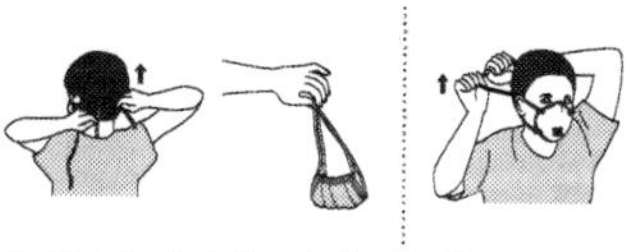

4. WASH HANDS OR USE AN ALCOHOL-BASED HAND SANITIZER IMMEDIATELY AFTER REMOVING ALL PPE

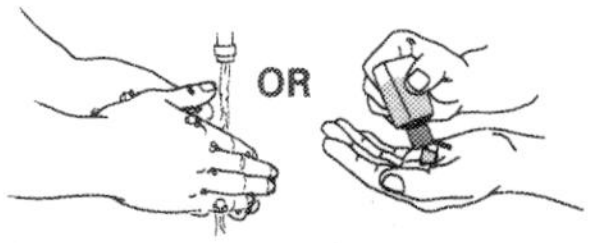

PERFORM HAND HYGIENE BETWEEN STEPS IF HANDS BECOME CONTAMINATED AND IMMEDIATELY AFTER REMOVING ALL PPE

CS250672-E

CHAPTER 5
Training

It is the employer's responsibility to ensure all employees have a safe and healthy work environment. General standards are regulated by OSHA. Specifically, OSHA standard 29 *CFR* 1910.132 explicitly requires employers to train employees in the safety aspects of their job. Training requirements not only require training on selection and use of PPE, but the standard also requires healthcare organizations to establish and audit for compliance training programs. In other words, your employer is mandated to train you, the employee, to recognize, avoid, lessen, or eliminate any potential workplace hazard or exposure to possible illness or injury. You must be trained to use any PPE to do your job, and your employer must provide you with that PPE and the training to use it properly.

The Problem of Noncompliance

In 1998, the Centers for Disease Control (CDC) published guidelines for infection control for healthcare personnel, placing emphasis on the need for a well-developed, comprehensive, and individualized approach to training of healthcare workers regarding how to protect themselves from potentially infectious diseases. It noted that workers are more likely to comply with an infection control program, to include use of PPE, if they understand why they need to wear it. It further points out that training programs should be tailored to meet the needs of workers based on their job category, risk of exposure, and literacy level.

Pro tip: Make it easy
During our Ebola training, my organization developed one standard training document. It was meant to train all employees in every job category. After the first training, which was attended by environmental services, laboratory technicians, registered nurses, physicians, and patient care technicians, the post-training evaluations indicated that staff had a difficult time following the material during the presentation. In other words, it was not user friendly. Fortunately, our organization had a focus on creating patient education materials that took into account people with lower levels of health literacy. We used similar principles like using pictorials, bullets instead of full sentences, lots of white space, and more demonstration.

Healthcare research bears out the need for coordinated, comprehensive, ongoing training of the healthcare worker concerning PPE in order to improve overall compliance. A survey of 653 hospital staff in five medical centers in Washington state found lack of knowledge by healthcare personnel about, and limited training on, recommended infection control practices and PPE usage as one of the rationales for lack of PPE compliance (Turnberg, Daniell, Seixas, Simpson, Van Buren, Lipkin, & Duchin, 2008).

Another study was able to demonstrate significant gaps in knowledge among healthcare workers concerning appropriate use of PPE and mechanism of infectious disease transmission in the healthcare setting. Most significant is the fact that healthcare workers failed to perform fit checks after putting on a respirator and did not get properly fit tested (Bryce, Forrester, Scharf, & Eshghpour, 2008).

In order for a hospital or healthcare organization to develop a successful, comprehensive, and safe PPE program designed to keep employees and patients safe from infections, it must proactively identify and fix workplace hazards before employees are injured or become ill. According to OSHA, any such program has as its foundation the following core elements:

- ❑ Leadership engagement and commitment
- ❑ Employee participation
- ❑ Hazard identification and assessment
- ❑ Hazard prevention and control
- ❑ Education and training
- ❑ Program evaluation and improvement

Many hospitals already have these elements in place to comply with The Joint Commission requirements for patient safety and becoming a high reliability organization. Thus, they are well poised to extend the same principles to successful employee safety programs such as PPE compliance.

Physicians have traditionally been the most difficult to train on the use of PPE for several reasons. The staff trainer is generally a nurse educator, who, in a traditionally hierarchical environment, may feel uncomfortable directing a superior. I personally watched this happen during training for donning and doffing for Ebola patients. Additionally, to my knowledge, after physicians complete residency training, there is no formal ongoing training regarding PPE purpose, use, selection, donning, doffing, and disposal. In many cases, visiting physicians are not employees of the healthcare organization, so mandatory OSHA training is not provided or required of them. Only during crisis or emerging infectious disease concerns will a concerted effort be made to include them. This has been borne out in a 2007 study about PPE compliance that concluded that physicians display poorer compliance than other categories of healthcare personnel (Manian & Ponzillo, 2007).

Keys to a Successful Training Program

First of all, workplace safety training programs must be ongoing and not just at new employee orientation. In building and implementing a comprehensive PPE training program, the following need to be addressed:

- ❑ What PPE is necessary based on the potential exposure to the employee
- ❑ When PPE is necessary
- ❑ How to check if PPE is damaged
- ❑ How to properly put on, remove, and dispose of PPE
- ❑ How to properly care for and store PPE if reusable
- ❑ Limitations of the PPE, if applicable
- ❑ How to evaluate worker compliance with PPE use

After the fundamentals of the program have been established, it might be helpful for the trainer to consider the following factors when implementing the training program:

- ❑ **Focus on what's in it for the employee.** If the purpose of the training is unclear or appears to benefit the hospital or even the patients only, many workers will not take the subject matter seriously. For instance, it may be more effective to remind the healthcare worker that performing the fit check prior to entering the room of a patient with influenza will increase the chance of being healthy for their family. This might resonate with workers better than stating they are expected to follow organizational policy and procedures for airborne precautions.
- ❑ **Benefit vs. burden.** The personal benefit must overshadow the training/requirement's perceived inconvenience for that person. For instance, wearing a respirator mask can be burdensome, especially if the worker believes he or she will just have to run a simple errand in the patient's room and will only be a few seconds. Always bear in mind that for most adults, including informed healthcare workers, their focus will be about their personal health and safety, so training and ongoing coaching must have that focus.
- ❑ **Personal costs.** Point out the real consequences for noncompliance. Consequences will reinforce the message for the worker. Discuss the actual outcomes for your organization or for the healthcare environment. No one wants to believe they would intentionally cause something bad to happen to them or their family. Many healthcare workers consider their place of work an extension of their family, as they have many friends and family members in the same organization, or their

friends and family members use their organization for their healthcare needs.

Training should attempt to put emphasis on the short-term and long-term effects for the individual if the health and safety precautions are not taken seriously. For instance, studies have shown that healthcare workers are at higher than average risk for developing infection with tubercolosis (TB) and active TB disease (Bausasano, Nunn, Williams, Pivetta, Bugianim, & Scano, 2011).

The short-term effect of having to take TB prophylaxis is the psychological toll of wondering if one is infected. The long-term effects are many, one of which is having to take a medication for months and dealing with the potential side effects of that medication. According to a nurse I know, who had to take such prophylaxis, he eventually developed peripheral neuropathy and lost sensation in his fingertips. For months, he could not use a glass to drink from. Think of the other impacts, too: on working as a nurse and on family obligations. Another effective way to highlight the personal costs is to share the organization's data on actual number of exposures/injuries by year that can be linked back to inappropriate or lack of use of PPE.

In healthcare, because we have so much training to accomplish, we tend to create lengthy training programs with the intent of capturing all required content in one session. After all, we are busy folks, right? I caution against that. During our organization's Ebola virus disease preparedness training, I watched as the eyes of employees glazed over, and in time they lost interest in the topic. It was apparent they were oversaturated. It's not that they did not think the topic was important; it's just that the training sessions occurred during their shifts, and they were concerned about other things—such as who was medicating their patient while they were in class.

Needless to say, the training session failed to meet its goals. We knew this because when it came time for return demonstration, the majority of the participants could not put on or remove PPE without step-by-step coaching. Some even challenged the information as invalid. Interestingly enough, one of the key lessons learned was that participants were able to re-engage during the interactive portions of the training session. We know the average adult will retain only about 20 minutes of content presented during a 90-minute training session.

There are great resources readily available to assist with developing lesson plans for adult students. Check out the following link for one of my favorite resources: *http://adulted.about.com/od/teachers/a/coursedesign.htm*.

Behavioral Goals

The ultimate goal of training is to influence behavior. Healthcare workers must understand what behaviors they will be able to do after the training that they were not able to do before. For instance, selecting the appropriate PPE for a particular situation, or how to put on an N-95 respirator mask are important tasks they must know, as it can save their lives.

Training content must be sensitive to this important fact. Build in pauses every 20 minutes or so to allow for feedback and/or return demonstration. As much as possible, include real-life scenarios. Provide quick reference or pocket guides such as this one to reinforce course content and ensure participants know where to go for assistance after the training session.

When PPE compliance becomes a normal everyday expectation, the U.S. healthcare system will not have to go into overtime and full-scale panic each time it is faced with a potential pandemic situation. Compliance with PPE should become a natural part of doing business for the healthcare worker.

In summary, there is no way around it: Healthcare employers must commit to providing repeated training and demonstrated competency for healthcare workers in the wearing and use of PPE. Everyone wins when the organization adopts a successful PPE training program.

References

Bausasano, I., Nunn, P., Williams, B., Pivetta, E., Bugianim, M., & Scano, F. (2011). "Tuberculosis among healthcare workers: Emerging infectious diseases." Vol.17, No. 3. *www.cdc.gov/eid.*

Bryce, E., Forrester, L., Scharf, S., & Eshghpour, M. (2008). What do healthcare workers think? A survey of facial protection equipment user preferences. *Journal of Hospital Infection,* 68(3), 241–247.

Manian, F.A., & Ponzillo, J.J. (2007). Compliance with routine use of gowns by healthcare workers (HCWs) and non-HCW visitors on entry into the rooms of patients under contact precautions. *Infection Control and Hospital Epidemiology,* 28(3), 337–340.

Turnberg, W., Daniell, W., Seixas, N., Simpson, T., Van Buren, J., Lipkin, E., & Duchin, J. (2008). Appraisal of recommended respiratory infection control practices in primary care and emergency department settings. *American Journal of Infection Control,* 36(4), 268–275.

CHAPTER 6

Promoting Safety Coaches

Changing behavior is a fundamental step in developing a culture of safety in any healthcare organization. About 40% of a healthcare organization's operating budget consists of human resources. Why not capitalize on this and use a human resources approach to improve safety practices? I recommend use of employees' knowledge to best gain buy-in by having them make inspections, hold safety training, coach their peers, and help to investigate accidents/errors when they are identified.

Unit-based safety coaches can act as valuable liaisons between staff and leadership to identify, address, and eliminate potential or real patient safety risks or concerns in particular PPE compliance.

Set annual targets, review what has been accomplished, and decide on new objectives or additional training requirements until the organization has hardwired safe PPE practices.

Unit- or department-based safety coaches just may be the link to ensuring staff and patient safety and improving compliance with PPE.

What Is a Safety Coach?

A robust safety coach program is believed to be key in reinforcing error-prevention practices and facilitating the spread of reliable, consistent, expected PPE selection and use to reduce harm to staff, patients, visitors, and employees. The safety coach's responsibilities include:

- ❑ Helping to teach and support colleagues in safe practices
- ❑ Encouraging open communication about PPE safety at all levels
- ❑ Identifying and sharing safety improvement opportunities and building accountability
- ❑ Promoting open communication and awareness of PPE selection and use protocols
- ❑ Acting as a role model
- ❑ Assisting with peer training and peer coaching at the unit/department level
- ❑ Conducting unit audits

Attributes of a safety coach include the following:

- ❑ A person who goes the extra mile
- ❑ Someone who feels comfortable providing feedback to others and is practiced in the art of skillful confrontation
- ❑ One who is passionate about safety
- ❑ A colleague who is seen as a top performer among peers and is well respected by all categories of staff
- ❑ Someone who has a questioning attitude

Resources necessary to support safety coaches:

- ❑ Executive sponsorship from the C-suite
- ❑ Time commitment from the following key stakeholders:

- — VP performance improvement
- — VP risk management
- — Physician champions
- — Infection prevention professionals
- — Unit-based safety coaches

- ❑ Dedicated meeting time (monthly, preferably, and not while assigned to regular duties)
- ❑ Meeting space
- ❑ Administrative support

Pro tip: Make it fun and rewarding to be a safety coach!
You can offer perks such as an identification badge with the title of Safety Coach or Safety Champion, public recognition at meetings, and public recognition on the organization's website and/or newsletters. Identify a few of your "super coaches" to be mentors to others. Invite them to attend or speak at outside educational events whenever possible.

The good news is that this model works for all other areas of safety focus once established. Safety coaches can be deployed to the organization's other safety initiatives such as hand hygiene.

Measuring Success

Healthcare organizations always seem to want to tout measures of success for any program implementation. Given that resources will need to be applied to any meaningful comprehensive safety coach program, it is likely that the organization would want to follow outcome measures, such as:

- ❑ Increase in Agency for Healthcare Research and Quality (AHRQ) or other culture of safety survey ratings
- ❑ Increase in PPE compliance on audits, particular in high-risk areas such as emergency department, obstetrics, critical care, etc.
- ❑ Decrease in employee exposure/injury events
- ❑ Decrease in hospital-acquired infection rates

Skillful Confrontation

In order for safety coaches to be successful, they must be able to engage in skillful confrontations. Skillful confrontation is the act of holding someone accountable for violated expectations or unacceptable performance through candid and respectful dialogue in such a way that problems are resolved, performance improves, and the relationship remains intact.

It may be helpful to create an unsafe action algorithm. I often witness staff enter an enhanced contact isolation room with gowns open in the back and hanging by their shoulder, leaving the upper body exposed. In their minds, they did don a gown. In 2015, I witnessed an emergency room technician with 20 years of experience start an intravenous line. He had gloves on but the two index fingers were torn off. When I asked why, the response was he needed to be able to feel the vein. Upon closer observation, the employee was wearing a glove size that was slightly too large. I mentioned this to the charge nurse who responded “we know, we’ve said something in the past, but the behavior has not changed, so we stopped trying to address the unsafe practice.”

We have all witnessed an unsafe practice by a coworker. We knew we should say something, but for some reason, we choke and simply walk away. Have you ever found yourself about to confront someone about inappropriate use of PPE only to start feeling nervous and apprehensive? When you experience this feeling, try telling yourself the positive reasons you should interject. Think of it as a normal conversation such as passing along a laboratory report (a statement of fact).

Some of the reasons healthcare workers passively stand by and witness breaches of appropriate PPE use without confrontation are:

- ❑ Fear of appearing to be picky, annoying, or a know-it-all
- ❑ Fear about the possible consequences with someone they see every day
- ❑ Fear that it may offend
- ❑ Thought that it may not be their place to speak
- ❑ Hope that someone else would do it
- ❑ Thought that they don't have the confidence or skill

Steps to Skillful Confrontation

Create a safe space and be sure your motives are to create a safer workplace instead of to criticize:

- ❑ Remain calm
- ❑ Be considerate and compassionate
- ❑ Don't assume the listener knows the correct procedures and adopt an attitude of curiosity

- ❑ Try to understand the other person's perspective
- ❑ Make sure your actions reinforce your words

Use the following three-step strategy called "describing the gap" to help make confrontations between colleagues more effective (Patterson, Grenny, McMillan, & Switzler, 2005).

- ❑ Describe what you see
- ❑ Describe what was expected versus what was observed
- ❑ Ask about the "gap" between the two

For example, "I notice you don't wear gloves when drawing blood, and the expectation is that we do. I'm curious why you don't."

Or: "I notice you don't wipe down the machine after using it." The question (Why not?) is implied.

Since you will be taking something away, give something back. Proposing options helps the other person see a way out, and it also signals respect. You could say something like, "I see those gloves you are wearing are too large; may I get the correct size for you?"

All staff are equal when discussing PPE safety concerns. It is important for there not to be hierarchy, real or perceived, as line staff will not confront peers or providers.

References

Patterson, K., Grenny, J., McMillan, R., & Switzler, A. (2005). *Crucial confrontations: Tools for resolving broken promises, violated expectations, and bad behavior.* New York: McGraw Hill.

For more information, check out the following link:

www.apic.org/Resource_/TinyMceFileManager/Topic-specific/Ebola_Readiness_Poll_Results_FINAL.pdf

CHAPTER 7
Conclusion

It is important to note that every healthcare organization has the responsibility and obligation to complete a risk assessment of its own organization to determine the appropriate PPE to be used by its workers. This risk assessment should look at the potential workplace hazards and likelihood of exposure. There should be clearly written and easily accessible standard operating procedures (SOPs) on the selection, use, storage, and decontamination (if reuse is allowed). Additionally, each organization should ensure ongoing training on how to select and wear the individual types of PPE.

To really drive the changes we need in healthcare, we need to adopt the strategies used around hand hygiene. You cannot walk into any healthcare organization now and not see signs of their emphasis on improving hand hygiene compliance, from readily available alcohol-based hand sanitizers to cough etiquette stations to hand hygiene compliance data. This focused effort to educate, train, monitor compliance, provide the required resources, and communicate openly can be attributed to the improvements we've seen with hand hygiene compliance.

Work-related injuries such as those resulting from accidental exposures can prevent healthcare workers from performing the job they love: caring for patients. Their lives are disrupted, and in some cases, exposures may even cause them to change careers. This then affects their role in society, their identity, and their socioeconomic status.

For employers, PPE compliance plays a major role in the prevention of occupational injuries and illnesses among healthcare workers, resulting in reducing days away from work, increasing job ability and task completion, and ensuring a healthier workforce which leads to better staffing ratios (ensuring a viable healthcare staff-to-patient ratio, etc.). Healthcare is one of the fastest growing sectors of the U.S. economy. Bureau of Labor statistics project this sector will add 5.6 million jobs during the next decade. Healthcare has added 559,000 jobs since the beginning of the recession in December 2007. Employment in healthcare is projected to continue to grow, which is even more reason for healthcare employers to make a concerted effort to instill good, consistent practices around PPE with their employees. A natural extension of a hospital's healing mission is to take measures to protect their workers' health and mitigate risk related to noncompliance with PPE use.

Notes

Notes

Quiz

Here's your chance to test your knowledge about what you've learned in this book. It's also a way for your employer to keep track of your training. When you're done, you can compare your answers by consulting the answer key on p. 61.

1. **Which of the following are steps to take when donning a face mask?**
   a. Place the mask over your nose, mouth, and chin
   b. Fit flexible nosepiece over nose bridge
   c. Secure on head with ties or elastic
   d. All of the above

2. **Which of the following is an example of the responsibilities of a safety coach?**
   a. Helping to teach and support their colleagues in safe practices
   b. Ensuring they are on call for emergency surgery
   c. Promoting open communication and awareness of PPE selection and use protocols
   d. Both A and C

3. **True or false: Sterile gowns are only necessary for performing invasive procedures, such as inserting a central line.**
   a. True b. False

4. **Which of the following is NOT a consideration when selecting proper PPE?**
   a. Durability of the PPE for the task
   b. Category of isolation precautions
   c. Color coordination with eye color
   d. Proper fitting of your mask and gloves

5. **All of the following are examples of reasons healthcare workers passively stand by and witness breaches of appropriate PPE EXCEPT:**
   a. Fear that it may offend someone
   b. Wanting to look good for the boss
   c. Fear about the possible consequences of speaking up
   d. Hope that someone else will do it

6. **True or false: When removing PPE after potential exposure to Ebola, healthcare workers should rely on the protocols they have memorized.**
   a. True b. False

7. **Which of the following are ways that creating a safety coach program can help employees improve PPE compliance?**
   a. Investigate accidents and errors
   b. Hold safety training sessions
   c. Help make safety inspections
   d. All of the above

8. **True or false: If you wear gloves when treating a patient, there is no need to wash your hands.**
   a. True b. False

9. **Which of the following are considerations to follow when doffing any PPE?**
   a. Assume that any surface in the patient's room could be contaminated
   b. Anyone wearing prescription eyeglasses should make sure the glasses are not contaminated when he or she removes PPE
   c. Gloves should always come off first
   d. Both A and B

10. **True or false: General Patton is credited with inventing the first respirator.**
    a. True b. False

This is to certify that I have read and understood the material in *The PPE Handbook for Healthcare Facilities.*

Name: ____

Date: ____

Answer Key

1. d. All of the above
2. d. Both A and C
3. a. True
4. c. Color coordination with eye color
5. b. Wanting to look good for the boss
6. b. False. The observer should use a checklist to avoid forgetting any steps in the process.
7. d. All of the above
8. b. False. Gloves do not replace the need for excellent hand washing or hand sanitizing with an alcohol-based sanitizer.
9. d. Both A and B
10. b. False. The painter Leonardo da Vinci is credited with inventing the first respirator.